YOUR KNOWLEDGE HAS VALUE

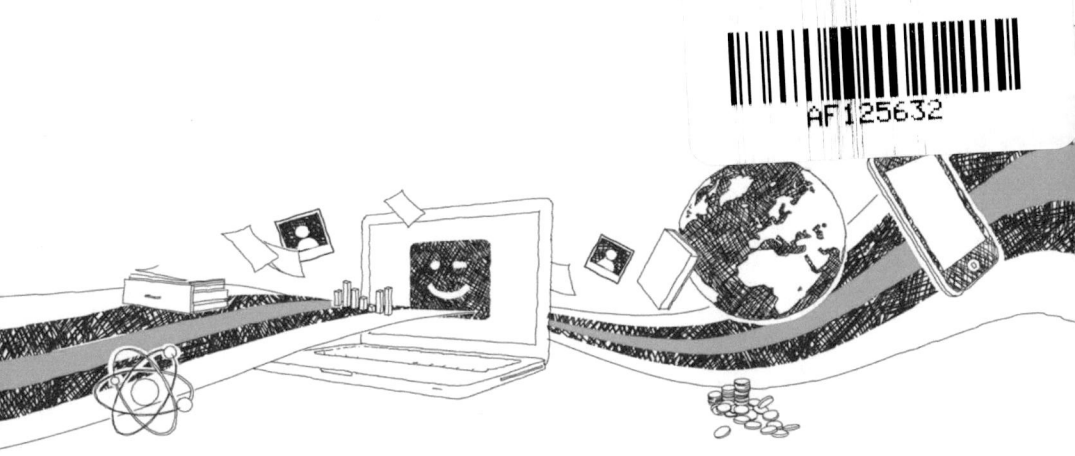
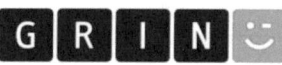

Bibliographic information published by the German National Library:

The German National Library lists this publication in the National Bibliography; detailed bibliographic data are available on the Internet at http://dnb.dnb.de .

Imprint:

Copyright © 2015 GRIN Verlag, Open Publishing GmbH
Print and binding: Books on Demand GmbH, Norderstedt Germany
ISBN: 978-3-668-02104-4

This book at GRIN:

http://www.grin.com/en/e-book/303796/what-kind-of-provisions-regulate-the-access-to-arv-medicine-and-how-did

Anonym

What kind of Provisions regulate the Access to ARV Medicine and how did Thailand react?

GRIN Publishing

GRIN - Your knowledge has value

Since its foundation in 1998, GRIN has specialized in publishing academic texts by students, college teachers and other academics as e-book and printed book. The website www.grin.com is an ideal platform for presenting term papers, final papers, scientific essays, dissertations and specialist books.

Visit us on the internet:

http://www.grin.com/

http://www.facebook.com/grincom

http://www.twitter.com/grin_com

Table of Contents

I. Introduction

The Human Immunodeficiency Virus, short called HIV, targets the human immune system and weakens the surveillance and defense system against infections. Infected people become gradually immunodeficient, while the virus destroys and impairs the function of immune cells. The Immune function is typically measured by the CD4 cell count. The most advanced stage of HIV is the Acquired Immunodeficiency Syndrome (AIDS).

HIV is a major public health issue, since it is the "world's most leading infectious killer" (WHO, 2014). Until today, no cure for HIV was found, but treatment with antiretroviral (ARV) drugs can help to control the virus. In a standard antiretroviral therapy (ART) are at least three antiretroviral drugs combatant to suppress the HIV virus and stop the progression of the disease.[1] In 2013 around 12.9 million people are receiving ART globally, of which 11.7 million were in low- and middle-income countries.

In 2010 the United Nations agreed to achieve a coverage of 15 million people on treatment worldwide by 2015 (United Nations, 2011) and most countries are aspiring to expand treatment access to around 80 percent of those in need, but this target has not been met on a global scale since the current coverage is at 65 percent.

Although it is well tried to achieve universal access to ARV drugs various trade laws make it harder to prevent everybody in need with medication. Further on, the behaviour of pharmaceutical companies play a big role for the access of ARVs.

It is to be said that I am going to focus my work on the TRIPS Agreement which was established in 1995, the trips agreement as 5 broader issues but I am going to concentrate on the protection of intellectual property rights, since this issue affects the access to HIV medication world wide. and the role of generic drugs. Ongoing, I will show off how Thailand reacted regarding TRIPS and how they used the flexibilities of it.

---

[1] A person should go under ART with a CD4 count less than 350 cells/mm3

II. Provisions that regulate the Access to ARVs

The TRIPS Agreement

The Agreement on Trade-Related Aspects of Intellectual Property Rights (TRIPS) sets the guideline to protect intellectual property worldwide, nowadays. It took in place on January, 1st 1995 and ties all members of the World Trade Organization[2] (WTO).

TRIPS sets a minimum standard of protection for intellectual property rights including patents, copyright, trademarks and industrialized designs (including medicine) it is enforced through the national legislation. These standards include that the protection of a patent was given at a minimum of 20 years beginning from the registration date. The patents can be given to products and processes. The question what is rather be protected by a patent is determined by the countries. The TRIPS Agreement does not define terms, like deciding whether a new combination (two ore more molecules are getting combined in one pill) or a new formulation (producing a pill version of a drug that once came as a powder) justifies for a twenty-year patent. These two terms a a privilege for the countries to decide because they are not determined by the WTO texts. Having that in mind, countries should determine what deserves a pharmaceutical patent, knowing there own economic and social situations[3] (MSF, 2011). It is also agreed in the TRIPS Agreement that transitional periodsare necessary for states to react and prepare. Industrialized countries got one year to implement TRIPS (until 1996) while developing countries got five years (until 2000) and least developed countries were given eleven years (until 2006). During the term of a patent the 'Bolar exemption' applies.

Bolar exemption:

In the TRIPS Article 30 is a limited exceptions to the rights commissioned to the patent holder. The most common exception to exclusive rights of the patent holder in the pharmaceutical context is referred as the 'Bolar provision[4] / Bolar exemption' . The 'Bolar exemption' allows interested (mainly generic) manufacturers to research and develop a new product before the patent expires.

---

[2] The WTO was established in 1995, it followed from the Uruguay Round and superseded GATT as an international Organization. Currently there are 160 members of the WTO of which 117 are developing countries ore separate customs. It is the umbrella organization of GATT,GATS and TRIPS. There main aim is to reduce trade barriers, liberalist the international trade and to protect customers and prevent the spread of diseases (WTO, 2013)

[3] A few governments like Brazil, India and Thailand have done that. (MSF, 2011)

[4] The name refers to a court case in the US, "Roche Products Inc. vs. Bolar Pharmaceutical Co. which dealt with this type of exception. (Jakarta, 2000)

This is important regarding the submission of information and samples to the regristration authorities. The purpose behind this is to get an approval of the generic drug before the patents expiration date to ensure that a generic drug can come onto the market shortly. (Nana K. Poku, Alan Vhiteside & Bjorg Sandkjaer, 2007 : 202)

Originally TRIPS was claimed to simulate the transfer of technology, to encourage foreign investments and to strengthen the research and development of new innovations, especially in least developed countries. Since the TRIPS agreement has a huge impact on generic drug production and controls in some ways the drug prices and tariffs and duties some analysts argued that TRIPS would decrease the health care system and strengthen monopolies. "The balance between the private interests of the patent holder and the larger interests of society is severely skewed" (MSF, 2011).

In 2001, at the annual conference of the WTO in Doha, the countries recognized the gravity of the imbalance regarding public health problems especially in developing and least developed countries. The Doha Declaration advocates countries rights to use TRIPS sponsorships like compulsory licenses or parallel impression to avoid patent barriers and promote access to medicine. A huge achievement of the meeting was to extend the transition period for least developed countries to another ten years (from 2006 to 2016). Especially the US supported by the EU, Japan, Switzerland and Canada[5] intended on preserving the protection of intellectual property rights, while Brazil and India[6] tried to strength the health safeguards. In the end the WTO agreed that:

"The TRIPS Agreement does not and should not prevent members from taking measures to protect public health"[7] (WHO, n.d.).

It has a few provisions under it, they can be used to avoid high drug prices charged by patent owners but it is each country can decide by themselves wether or not they want to convert those safeguards into their national law or not. Those provisions are the compulsory license, voluntary license and parallel imports. I will explain all three of them more in the following.

---

5 all of them are developed countries
[6] both are least developed countries
[7] §§ 4-6

Compulsory licensing

A compulsory license is an authorization granted by the government without the permission of the patent holder. Every country has the right to file a compulsory license either through their own patent law or through the TRIPS Agreement. TRIPS does not set the standards of the grounds or reasons for granting such a license but countries can only use the grounds given by their national legislation. However, TRIPS wants the states to regulate those conditions corresponding to the TRIPS Agreement Article f9 31.

Grounds for compulsory licenses have been specified by countries in many different ways, for example public health reasons, instance emergency situations, epidemics, public non-commercial use, to find a solution for anti-competitive practices or to protect the environment. Since it is a national law decision, which ground is going to be chosen there is a lot of flexibility given[8].

A compulsory license does not subduct the rights of a patent holder, it simply limits the rights more than before. TRIPS specifies the conditions that need to be applied, once a country wants to grant a compulsory license. An important point is that every case needs to be treated individually. The first step is in general to obtain a license from the patent holder, a voluntary license, on adequate terms.[9] In case of a national emergencies or other circumstances of extreme urgency is no need to file for a voluntary license at first, this is the only instance when the TRIPS Agreement links directly to a compulsory license to save time. Even if a compulsory license is granted through the government the licensees still have to pay a royal fee to the patent holder. Nevertheless, it is to mention that such a few is significantly lower as a voluntary license fee and it still makes medicine more affordable to people than before.

The general case of a compulsory license is when the generic copy is produced mainly for the domestic market and not for the export. However, the 2001 Doha Ministerial Conference decided that this general case should be changed. Countries shall now obtain cheaper generic drugs elsewhere, if necessary. This change became legal on 30 August, in 2003[10]. From this point, generic copies made under a compulsory license can

---

[8] For example the German law states that a compulsory license can be filled in case of a reason of public interest. This description can be used in many ways.
[9] what is intended to be adequate depends on the national law
[10] this Decision is sometimes called Paragraph 6

be exported to countries that lack production capacity. Countries may have to change their national law to implement the new provision. (WTO, 2006)

In least developed countries the government does not have to grant for a compulsory license before 2016, since TRIPS does not implement before then. A compulsory license has to be granted in case a supplying country would export a generic drug that is patented in that country (WTO, 2006).

The problem of compulsory licenses is that pharmaceutical companies will try to subdue compulsory licenses, by threatening the government not to produce in their country anymore if they might issue a compulsory license. This means many countries do not even allow compulsory licenses in their national patent law, to avoid threats from pharmaceutical companies.

It is questionable if a small country should grant a compulsory license, since their domestic market could be to small to be rentable. Another negative effect is that the reputation of a country could get damaged due granting a compulsory license. It was even worse before the Doha declaration, when it was decided that countries could put down their own ground rules for issuing a compulsory license rather than announcing an epidemic health crisis. But even now the word will spread once a compulsory license is issued. A damaged reputation of a country could lead to a decrease of the economic[11].

Voluntary licensing

A voluntary license can be granted by a patent holder to other manufacturers, in this case the patent holder would allow others to produces a generic drug in exchange for royalty payments.

Nevertheless, the patent holder could rise conditions or limitations on voluntary licenses through negotiations. Especially in the HIV context, pharmaceutical companies could argue that exportation can only be regional and exportation to developed markets in the north are prohibited at all times, even under parallel importation rules. Also a patent holder can decide how many manufactures will be allowed to get a voluntary license (mainly it is just one company), this is also called an exclusive voluntary license. It is to

---

[11] The trade with this country would shrink, either import or/and export, also the tourisms into this country would go down.

6

distinguish whether it is an exclusive or non-exclusive basis on which the licenses is granted. An exclusive basis means the the patent holder can put down rules, like 'how many manufacturers are allowed to produce the generic'. A voluntary license on a non-exclusive basis means that everyone is allowed to produce the generic. In both terms will be a substantial price reduction because of the voluntary license.

However, it could happen that because of those prohibitions from certain pharmaceutical companies, patients would not benefit from the lowest price possible, nor is it that the access to medicine worldwide is increasing.

Also a well known fact is that pharmaceutical companies are unlikely to agree on a voluntary license, because that would mean they had to give up their monopolies which would implement a lost of welfare.

Parallel importing

Parallel imports are also referred to the 'grey market' of imports. They often take place in case of a difference in the pricing of the same product - it can be the brand name or the generic drugs - in different markets.

The TRIPS Agreement specifically says that the procedure of parallel imports can not be challenged under the WTO dispute settlement system, which leads it to be a national concern or policy.

Using parallel imports can lead to a price reduction of medicine through competition. Nevertheless, it can also have a huge influence on the negotiations of staged pricing regimes with pharmaceutical companies. In case a private pharmaceutical company would agree to charge a low price on a drug in poor countries, it is going to ask for assurance that the government would import the cheaper product into the more wealthy country market to try undercutting profits. Since parallel imports are not regulated in TRIPS, pharmaceutical industries will try to blank parallel imports by threatening the government not to sell any drugs at all, if parallel import is possible (WHO, n.d.).

According to the ASEAN[12] Workshop on the TRIPS Agreement and its impact on pharmaceuticals is it possible that parallel import in developing countries will lead to an

---

[12] ASEAN stands for Associaton of Southeast Asian Nations and is an international NGO

increased counterfeit and substandard products in the pharmaceutical market, which will automatically lead to an negative impact for customers (Jakarta, 2000).

TRIPS Plus "TRIPS Plus is going even further than TRIPS" (MSF, 2011).
It is not a multi-lateral agreement like TRIPS. It puts many developing countries under pressure to apply even tougher conditions in their own patent laws than they are required by the TRIPS Agreement, the so called TRIPS Plus provisions. They are seen as bilateral free trade agreements. Legally countries are not indebted to implement TRIPS Plus but many countries, such as Brazil, China or Central American state have had no chance then to adopt those provisions to their trade agreements, since they were put under pressure from the United States of America or the European Union (Nana K. Poku, Alan Vhiteside & Bjorg Sandkjaer, 2007 : 208).

Under the TRIPS Plus provisions a country may be forced to raise the IPRs to a higher level of protection than under TRIPS, such as being forcefully required to implement more extensive levels and standards of IPR protection. If a country ignores a point on the TRIPS agreement, it could lead forward to TRIPS Plus. Examples of the TRIPS Plus provision are extending the term of a patent even longer than the 20-year minimum, provisions that may limit the use of compulsory licenses or restriction of generic competition.

One well known provision is the 'data exclusivity provision', it refers to exclusive right given for pharmaceutical test data which is submitted by generic manufacturers to get market authorization. This basically means that informations regarding the efficiency or safety of a drug is kept confidential, over a period of time[13]. This provision prohibits to put a generic drug on the market right after the patent expired because they have either sit out the exclusivity period or going under extensive long-timed clinical trials to prove the safety and efficiency of a generic drug. TRIPS Plus provisions are pushed as a part of free trade agreements between developed and developing countries (MSF, 2011). Especially the USA and EU tried to enforce stronger patent rights by threatening to impose sanctions on countries that did not follow their bilateral contracts.

---

[13] there is no special period determined, but it is mostly around 5 to 10 years

8

III. Which provision has been applied? Case study Thailand - granting a compulsory license

The military-backed government in Thailand issued a compulsory license to the Government Pharmaceutical Organisation (GPO) on 29 November in 2006, for the Mercks's HIV/AIDS drug 'Efavirenz' and in the beginning of 2007 the 'Kaletra' HIV Drug. Their main goal was to cut growing costs, regarding to health care by encouraging the import and production of generic versions of the drug. The compulsory license was endorsed by the Clinton Foundation, 22 US senators, the WHO and UNAIDS. (Baron, 2008)

However, the compulsory license came with a few terms. The GPO has to pay 5 percent of the total sale value of the imported or locally-produced drug (Bridges, 2006). Another term was that only 200.000 people would be allowed the generic drug per year. The compulsory license was valid through 31 December in 2011.The government decided to issue a compulsory license after more and more people got infected with HIV and they could not provide free medicine for everyone as they committed since the prices for ARVs were to high. Also negotiations with pharmaceutical companies about lowering their medicine prices failed. It turned out that the pharmaceutical companies were only willing to negotiate with the government to buy time for themselves, time in which the price of the medicine will not decrease.

After the compulsory license was granted, a positive outcome was seen after only a short period of time, after just two years 30.000 HIV infected people were now covered with ARVs (before the compulsory license it has been 5000) on first-line-treatment and 5000 in second-line-treatment (before 300) (MSF, 2009).

Although, it seems that a compulsory license only comes with benefits it takes a lot of courage for a country like Thailand to issue one. Many developing countries are simply to afraid to grant a compulsory license because of measures from pharmaceutical companies and from countries where pharmaceutical lobbies are stronger, the reputation of a country, a potential economic crisis and various other reasons. As mentioned in an upper paragraph, pharmaceutical companies could simply refuse to produce or sell in markets where strict controls or provisions like compulsory licenses could be possible. Especially in Thailand pharmaceutical lobbies from stronger countries reacted to their action, the US government put Thailand on the 'US trade-blacklist'. Another concern is that a country which is granting a compulsory license could destroy their image because of the press (also mentioned in an upper paragraph).

The case Thailand showed that many of those fears were proved invalid. Although, Thailand was on the blacklist by the US government, the overall trading numbers did not drop like they were feared to and so the economy was still strong and growing (MSF, 2009).

The Government of Thailand went even a step further, in 2010 and extended the compulsory license for Efavirenz and Kaletra as well until their patents would expire[14] (Avert, n.d.).

All in all, the Thai story is a huge success story and should give a great example for other developing countries, in need for cheaper ARVs, to issue a compulsory license

IV. Conclusion

TRIPS is an important provision regarding the access to medicine. In the beginning of TRIPS it started out as an agreement only trying to protect intellectual property rights. On the one hand, TRIPS established to protect those IPs, but with the positive outcome of encouraging individuals to be creative, innovative and even brave enough to invest in new technologies and new formulas for medicine. On the other hand, TRIPS misleads the owners of a patent to exploit their powerful position and to strengthen monopolies, which leads to an imbalance between helping people in need an getting profits for pharmaceutical companies.

The Doha Declaration was one step in the right direction, but still not enough to avoid pharmaceutical companies or developed countries to use their 'power' against least developed or/and developing countries. The welfare of countries or/and companies should not be more important than global health. The fact that wealthier countries have such an influence on poorer countries should be eliminated. The only way to achieve this, is for least developed countries and developing countries to push implemented safeguards, such as compulsory licensing, threw.

---

[14] Efavirenz patent did expire January 2012 and Kaletra in December 2016

TRIPS it not just a bad thing, it is important to protect IPs, otherwise big pharmaceutical companies would not try to invent new technologies and medicine. However, protection intellectual property rights should stop, or get less important, as soon as public health is in risks or neglected.

It is obvious that although the access to ARVs has improved during the years through different measures, like demanding to start ART with a CD4 count by 300 cells/mm3 rather than 500 cells/mm3 by the WTO or to encourage especially least developed countries to issue a compulsory license, voluntary license or implement parallel imports during the Doha, it is not enough to reach universal access. Especially regardingcompulsory licensing is more needed than the common situation. It should be illegal for pharmaceutical companies to put pressure onto the government in they try to grant a compulsory license. The WHO should also take more responsibility in this subject matter, since they failed from the beginning on. They are a big player regarding global health and should act like that.

All in all, a perfect balance between the protection of patients and patents can only be achieved, if all players find a compromise, which they all are satisfied with.

List of References

Avert n.d., *compulsory licensing*. Available from: http://www.avert.org/hiv-drugs-patents-legislation.htm. [02/28/2015]

Baron, David 2008, *Compulsory Licensing, Thailand, and Abbott Laboratories.î* Stanford Graduate School of Business Case P-66.

Bridges 2006, *Thailand Issues Compulsory Licence For Patented AIDS Drug.* Available from: http://www.ictsd.org/bridges-news/bridges/news/thailand-issues-compulsory-licence-for-patented-aids-drug. [02/26/2015]

Jakarta 2000, *Report of an ASEAN Workshop on the TRIPs Agreement and its Impact on Pharmaceuticals.* Available from: http://apps.who.int/medicinedocs/pdf/h1459e/h1459e.pdf. [02/22/2015].

Medicine Sans Frontieres 2009, *Audio: Compulsory licensing in Thailand.* Available from: http://www.msf.org/article/audio-compulsory-licensing-thailand. [02/28/2015]

Medicines Sans Frontieres 2011, *TRIPS, TRIPS Plus and Doha.* Available from http://www.msfaccess.org/content/trips-trips-plus-and-doha .[02/20/2015].

Nana K. Poku, Alan Vhiteside & Bjorg Sandkjaer 2007, *AIDS and Governance.*

United Nations 2011, *Implementation of the Declaration of Commitment on HIV/AIDS and the Political Declaration on HIV/AIDS.* Available from: http://daccess-dds-ny.un.org/doc/UNDOC/LTD/N11/367/84/PDF/N1136784.pdf?OpenElement .[02/20/2015].

World Health Organization 2014, *10 Facts on HIV/AIDS.* Available from: http://www.who.int/features/factfiles/hiv/en/. [02/19/2015].

World Trade Organisation 2006, *Compulsory licensing of pharmaceuticals and TRIPS.* Available from: https://www.wto.org/English/tratop_e/trips_e/public_health_faq_e.htm .[02/22/2015].

World Health Organization 2014, *HIV/AIDS Fact sheet N°360.* Available from: http://www.who.int/mediacentre/factsheets/fs360/en/. [02/19/2015].

World Health Organisation n.d., *THE DOHA DECLARATION ON THE TRIPS AGREEMENT AND PUBLIC HEALTH.* Available from: http://www.who.int/medicines/areas/policy/doha_declaration/en/ .[21/02/2015].

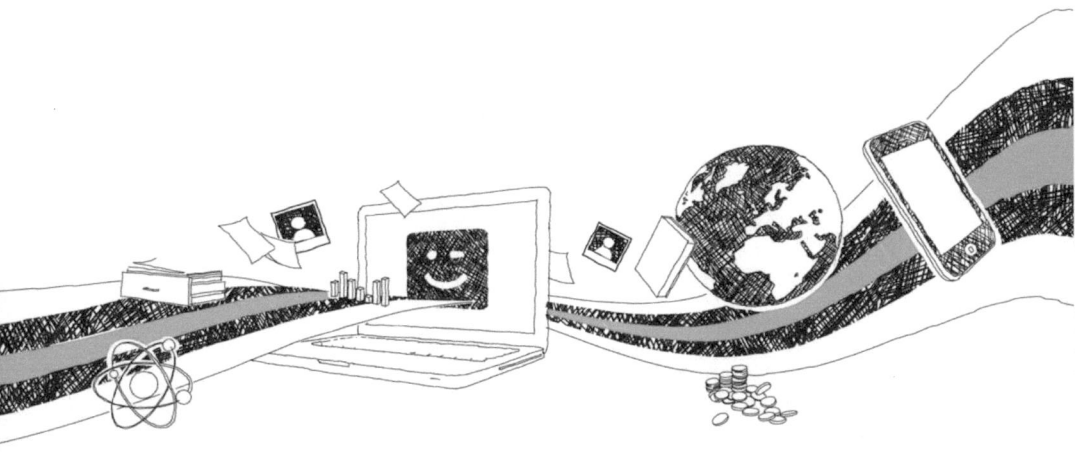
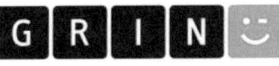